BRAIN, BODY & BEING™

Five Secrets for Achieving Authentic Health & Happiness

by

Dr. Jay Kumar

Published in the United States of America
ISBN: 9781619849907

Made in the USA
San Bernardino, CA
07 February 2017

Contents

A Secret That Will Transform Your Life

Imagine waking up genuinely healthy and happy.
Imagine feeling full of vitality, serenity and joy.
Imagine experiencing a deeper sense of love, purpose and meaning.
    Why not begin this journey today!
    We all want to feel younger, be happier and live longer. Thousands of books hype the latest way to lose weight, firm your abs and get rich. The implication is that shedding pounds, toning muscles and fattening your bank account will make one happy. So, how is this book on how to get healthy and happy any different?
    For starters, it's based on the premise that what you think, how you feel and even how you breathe have a greater impact on the quality of your health and happiness than any workout, vitamin or diet. As you'll discover as you read on, this isn't wishful thinking or a New Age concept, it's based on cutting-edge research from neuroscience, cognitive psychology and mind-body medicine.
    In these pages, I'll share with you secrets that aren't widely known or understood by most health gurus, fitness experts or lifestyle celebrities. What I am about to share will make you view health and happiness in an entirely new light.
    Medical research now tells us that if your life is riddled with stress, fear and anxiety, you might accelerate the aging process in your DNA by as much as 600%! Put another way, for every year you live, stress tacks on an additional full six years than if you lived a life of minimal stress.
    Many of us struggle to exercise and eat right. But even if you succeed, those benefits are reduced if you routinely feel stressed, anxious and overwhelmed.

If this surprises you, you're not alone. You might even be the first among all your friends to discover this amazing fact.

But what if I told you how in as little as 10 to 15 minutes a day there are proven ways you could dramatically lower your level of stress. These tools will not only allow you to live longer, but they will boost your sense of happiness and improve your overall health.

I invite you to take this first step toward achieving authentic health and happiness today. I promise you won't regret it!

So How Can Brain, Body & Being™ Help Me?

It's only in the past 10 to 15 years since the advent of technology that allows doctors and researchers to peer directly inside the human brain in real-time without using a scalpel. Cutting-edge neural-imaging devices make it possible to explore the uncharted territory of the human brain. These discoveries are upending many long-held beliefs about human behavior, emotions and health.

For instance, it was thought that by the time we reach early adulthood, the human brain was fixed, immutable and rigid. The ability to acquire new tools and tasks, though still possible, was considered to be more difficult as we grew older.

It was once argued that while medication or therapy could help in changing human behavior in the treatment of depression and anxiety, such methods couldn't alter the fundamental neural structures of the brain. All of these limiting beliefs have fallen away in the past decade!

One recent revolutionary discovery—*neuroplasticity*—affirms that it is possible to "teach an old brain new tricks."

If you're not a scientist or doctor, why should you care about neuroplasticity? Because it may well prove to be the "Holy Grail" that allows us to experience long-lasting and authentic health and happiness.

What neuroscience has affirmed is that the brain is not fixed, but plastic and adaptable. This radical concept known as neuroplasticity explores how our thoughts, feelings, actions, attitudes and behaviors can physically alter our brain structure.

When you consciously change your thoughts, you physically change your brain—and your life!

Think of the neural pathways in the brain like a trail in the woods. The more you walk it, the more worn the path. In a similar manner, the thoughts and feelings that run through our heads form pathways. The more we feel overwhelmed, angry, shameful or depressed, neurons in the brain attach themselves, creating neural pathways that reinforce these thoughts. Ultimately, these neural pathways become our "default" response system in life.

Let's say your girlfriend decided to walk out or you botched an interview that would have boosted your career. Such events trigger previous situations where you felt abandoned or a sense of failure. Based on the existing neural pathways in your brain from the past, old-patterns of thought kick in, leading you to conclude: "I'm a loser! I always screw things up. Nobody loves me."

Neuroplasticity offers us hope! It suggests that whenever we encounter a new experience, we no longer have to travel down that familiar path of shame or regret. We now have a choice. Rather than falling back on the same patterns of thoughts and behavior, we have a new opportunity to respond to life in a way that promotes our health and happiness.

What I find most exciting is that when we make empowering choices, and develop new healthful habits, our brain imprints those changes. This can happen whether you're 19 or 91.

Neuroplasticity, in essence, states, "You become what you chronically think."

The more you choose to think, act and feel affirming thoughts, such as love, joy, forgiveness, gratitude and compassion, your brain will rewire itself to reflect those attributes. The more you do this, the stronger the connections in your brain. That's neuroplasticity in a nutshell.

It turns out, Abraham Lincoln had it right. "Most people are as happy as they make up their minds to be."

One frequent question that arises in my university course on "Happiness" is: "If nature allowed the human brain to be wired for happiness, why is it then that so many of us go through life feeling depressed, lonely or sad?"

My answer is that most of us have never been taught how to harness the brain's innate potential for happiness. We literally possess the ability to sculpt the brain to be happy or sad. This is no longer wishful thinking. It's actual science.

Happiness it turns out is a quality that we are all capable of wiring into the *brain*, experiencing in our *body* and manifesting in our *being*.

As a young adult, I frequently felt overwhelmed by stress and depression. I wish that at the time I had the tools and awareness to combat these feelings. After many years, studying in ashrams and Ivy League schools, I finally came upon my own answers as to how to achieve health and happiness.

I've created this book for one specific reason: to educate, empower and engage you in the revolutionary 21st-century science that shows us how to attain authentic health and happiness. These findings are what inspire me to teach these tools in college campuses and corporate boardrooms.

Just as we can strengthen our abs doing sit ups, we can also train our brain for health and happiness.

So what do I mean when I use the term: *Brain, Body & Being*™?

The *brain* is more than just the 3-pound mass of jelly-like tissue in our skull. In actuality, the brain comprises more than 100 billion neurons and other nerve cells. These neurons form part of the nervous system that runs down the spine and throughout every inch of our body. Neurons have most recently been discovered to be present in our heart and gut.[1] Collectively this larger "brain" enables information, thoughts and feelings to be transmitted throughout the body.

The *body* is more than just the external physical structure. It includes the totality of all the organs—the digestive, immune, circulatory, reproductive and other systems—as well as trillions of cells and DNA molecules. Why consider the body from this microscopic perspective? Because medical science can now prove that lowering stress, slowing down aging and improving our health occur at a genetic and cellular level.

But what's being? One's *being* encompasses the vast mental, emotional and spiritual terrain of thought, feelings, memory and consciousness. It is through our being that we express our love, joy, dreams and creativity. In short, it is our essence.

Here's the best part. All the tools you will ever need on this journey of personal transformation arise from within. There's no vitamin to buy, no gadget or equipment to purchase.

This is why I invite you to: "Engage Your *Brain*, Heal Your *Body*, and Transform Your *Being*." It's a sure path that will lead you to authentic health and happiness.

How Stress Sabotages Health & Happiness

A lot of us follow a healthy diet, exercise regularly and yet still feel burdened by stress, illness or sadness. Is it even realistic in this day and age to achieve authentic health and happiness? Yes!

Here's why. Consider something as simple as your breath. When you feel anxious or stressed, your breath becomes erratic, quick or shallow. This is caused by a mechanism in the brain's nervous system known as the stress-response.

Here's what I find fascinating about the stress-response? It works exactly the same whether you're being chased by a lion or stuck in a traffic jam! The brain can't distinguish between a "real" versus a "perceived" threat to one's survival. While the brain's automatic stress-response is vital in helping us to avoid actual danger, left unchecked, the stress-response has harmful effects such as suppressing one's digestion, immunity, sleep or sex-drive.

Put it in the simplest terms, stress is Enemy No. 1. In far too many lives, stress causes illness, exhaustion or sorrow.

Consider how many times a day your own stress response is activated. The kids act up, your boss behaves like a jerk or you learn your credit card bill is through the roof. In every one of these situations, even though there is no immediate danger to your physical survival, your stress-response is triggered.

The moment it kicks in, the *brain* immediately alerts your *body* to be on alert. Stress hormones cortisol and adrenaline are unleashed in your bloodstream. This flood of stress chemicals triggered by the brain into the body has a significant impact on your overall emotional, psychological and mental state of *being*.

Stress kills! Along with its related conditions it is the number one cause of death in the United States.[2] Stress not only threatens one's ability to be healthy and happy, studies show some 75% of Americans suffer from stress.

age 6x as fast. As mentioned earlier, stress has the potential to make us age as much as six times more quickly! Dr. Elizabeth Blackburn and her team at the UCSF Medical School won the 2009 Nobel Prize in Medicine by showing how chronic stress connects to premature aging by damaging our cells and DNA.[3]

We are a nation held hostage by stress. Instead of waging a "War on Terror," perhaps what we as a nation need is a "War on Stress." Stress keeps us trapped in survival mode. Think about it this way, if all your body's energy is depleted simply trying to survive, how can you ever expect yourself fully to thrive?

Before you throw in the towel and give up hope, here's some good news. While research tells us that stress accelerates aging and impairs our health, an increasing number of medical studies points out that our body is already equipped with natural ways to counter the harmful effects of stress.

I can't wave a magic wand and make all the sources of stress in your life disappear. No one can do that. What I can show you are tools, so that when faced with stress, you can engage the brain's *relaxation response.*

But how can you relax when you feel stressed? One route is the breath. There's an intimate connection between our breath and relaxation. More and more studies indicate that by simply slowing down and breathing into the lower belly, one can trigger the body's natural relaxation response. Deepen your breathing, and the *brain* activates the important vagus nerve, immediately stopping the release of harmful stress hormones. The result? "Feel-good" chemicals—dopamine, serotonin and oxytocin—are released into the *body*, shifting one's state of *being* from stress to serenity. What's even more amazing is that we can notice this shift happening in as little as ten seconds.

This isn't New Age thinking. It's science!

A 2009 report from the Harvard Medical School stated that patients, who practiced breathing exercises six times a week over a four-week period, had a 67% remission rate from chronic depression. [4] More clinical trials are offering similar results, championing the medical benefits of deep-belly breathing and other breathing exercises as on par with or even surpassing the efficacy of medication in the treatment of post-traumatic stress syndrome, bi-polar disorder, anxiety and insomnia.

*While I'm not suggesting anyone discontinue taking anxiety or depression meds, I do advocate breath work as a daily practice.

Dr. James S. Gordon, a clinical professor of psychiatry at the Georgetown University School of Medicine, wrote: "Slow, deep breathing is probably the single best anti-stress medicine we have."

Be forewarned: Slow, deep breathing may cause beneficial, long-lasting side effects, including increased happiness, optimism, health, calm, compassion, alertness and joy. Stress may be an inevitable fact of life, but it's how we respond to stress that matters.

Excessive stress damages DNA.

↓ good & Bad ways To get out of stress.

Secret 1 | Your Brain Wants You To Be Happy

No external conditions are required for happiness. Happiness is who you are! —Dr. Jay Kumar

That's right! We are wired to be happy. Even the Declaration of Independence boldly asserts that each one of us is endowed with "certain unalienable rights that among these are Life, Liberty and the pursuit of Happiness." Modern science, especially the cutting-edge fields of contemplative neuroscience and positive psychology, affirm this fundamental truth—we are not only *meant to* be happy, we are *wired to* be happy!

Contrary to what our society, media or culture wants us to believe, our species is not programmed for strife, conflict, fear and anxiety. While unpleasant feelings exist, we are in actuality, wired to feel healthy, happy and whole.

Let's explore why our brains are wired for happiness.

The human brain allows us to engage in distinct types of attention. One is a "voluntary or active" attention that enables us to focus our thoughts and energy on tasks that require concentration. "Involuntary or passive" attention, is something our brains do with little or no effort. Throughout the day the brain alternates between active and passive types of mental attention.

Notice the difference in your awareness when you're studying for an exam or working to meet a deadline versus when you are enjoying a sunset, listening to music or playing with your dog.

The first type of activity requires a hyper-focused state of attention or concentration on the immediate task at hand. By contrast, when we feel relaxed and not under pressure our brains are in a passive state of awareness that allows us to experience the fullness of the moment.

So why is this important? It turns out that prolonged activity of the brain in active-attention mode leads to "brain-fatigue," which makes us more prone to stress, anxiety, weight gain, low sex-drive, insomnia and accelerated aging. But the more we allow the brain to be in a state of passive-attention, the more we optimize health, longevity, relaxation, sleep, memory and happiness.

In our waking state, the brain waves associated with each of these two types of attention look different. When one is engaged in active attention the brain is predominantly in a beta wave state. When one is in a state of passive attention, the brain produces alpha waves. (Theta and delta wave states generally occur during sleep)

Don't get me wrong. There's nothing wrong with active attention. We need this beta wave activity when driving, playing sports or performing any task that requires focus and concentration. The problem arises when we spend too much of our day with our brain in this highly attuned beta wave state.

My advice here isn't to shirk responsibility, play hooky and hang out at the beach. What many people are surprised to discover is that spending time in a calm and soothing alpha wave state, replenishes the brain. This alpha wave state helps us to find greater inspiration and clarity, and we find ourselves able to accomplish more in less time than if we never took a break from the task at hand.

But how do brain waves tie in to our health and wellbeing? A growing wealth of research from medical institutions such as the UCLA Center for Psychoneuroimmunology points to a correlation between our brain waves and our general state of health and level of happiness.[5]

As you recall, a threat doesn't have to be real to be hazardous to one's health. When the brain is amped up from information overload it creates a frenetic beta wave state. This releases a flood of the stress hormones adrenaline and cortisol throughout the body. Your boss shoots you an email that she wants you ASAP in her office. She may want to commend you for landing a new client, but your brain is already inventing worst-case scenarios.

This is why it's so important to learn how to enter a relaxed alpha wave state so your thoughts don't needlessly take you down the path of dread and worry. Fortunately the brain is malleable and it can learn new behaviors. We not only possess a stress-response, but the brain also has a built-in relaxation response.

This is precisely why everyone has the potential to be happy and healthy. We are born with this "operating system" already installed in our brain. We just need to learn how to use it. While the breath is one very easy tool that switches on our innate relaxation-response, there are other equally effective means to promote our health and happiness.

Let's explore them.

↓ Happiness (vs) Pleasure

Secret 2 | Happiness Lasts, Pleasure Fades

Pleasure has a limited shelf life. Happiness has no expiration date! —Dr. Jay Kumar

It certainly was a big revelation in my life many years ago when I learned that pleasure and happiness are not the same. As an avowed "pleasure-seeker" in my younger years, I admit it took me some time to recognize how I confused happiness with pleasure.

While most of us strive to feel happy, many of us remain stuck on the path of pleasure. I concede that happiness is a vague term, personally defined, culturally relative and, in many ways, a social construct. But just because people confuse happiness with pleasure, the brain does not.

Think about the many ways we experience pleasure. We may enjoy gourmet food, making love, a bottle of Pinot Noir, a luxury cruise to Tahiti, a wild night out on the town, a shopping spree, Super Bowl tickets…. Now think about the things in life that bring you happiness: your children, your cat or dog, your partner or close friends.

Do you notice a difference between these two lists? Things that tend to bring us pleasure are all fleeting experiences. Once the feeling of pleasure is gone, we yearn for the next time we'll have it. Happiness, however, is a state that is independent of an external situation or experience. Happiness can even be triggered by a mere thought or memory.

While we likely would feel happy watching the sunset on a beach in Hawaii, if I asked you to recall the memory of viewing such a sunset, you would be able to trigger that same feeling of happiness.

Compare that with the pleasure of savoring a slice of hot apple pie à la mode. If asked to recall that experience, would you feel the same pleasure as when you actually ate it?

Think of it this way. Pleasure is a sensation. Happiness is a feeling. As I stated earlier, pleasure has a limited shelf life. Happiness has no expiration date!

Don't get me wrong. We need pleasure in our lives. Indeed, pleasure in limited doses is good for us. "Pleasure circuits" are built into the brain. When these pleasure areas of the brain are activated, the neurotransmitters dopamine and serotonin are released throughout the body. This is what triggers the sensation of euphoria and excitement, be it from an orgasm or online-gambling.

Pleasure is intimately connected to the brain's reward and gratification centers. This is how people become addicted to food, alcohol, tobacco, video games, sex, shopping, slot machines or even certain types of relationships. Each of these pursuits taps the pleasure centers in the brain. It's worth noting that the more we stimulate the brain's pleasure centers, the more of the actual thing is needed to experience the prior level of gratification.

Once we experience the excitement and thrill of a pleasurable situation, we tend to crave more of it. Consider the first blush of romance, when you're crazy about someone and can't wait for the next time you'll be together. That's the brain's pleasure center taking over.

Ironically, sometimes the more we experience something the less pleasurable it becomes. Consider how pleasurable it is taking that first bite of chocolate cake, and how much less satisfying it tastes once you've eaten two slices. Pleasure can also diminish the more we experience it.

The same is not true of happiness. While pleasure comes and goes, happiness is a feeling that is long lasting. Of course, some sources of our happiness—your kids, your spouse, your dog who devours a favorite pair of shoes—don't make us all that happy. Yet, in the long term, happiness outweighs short-term displeasure.

Think of happiness as an emotional and spiritual quality while pleasure is physical and sensory. The brain knows the difference! There are even separate areas of the brain that correspond to pleasure and happiness.

None of this is a fluke. There are evolutionary reasons for this. Indeed, pleasure supports human survival. First, there's the obvious reason. Procreation is fun! Pleasure is wired into our primal brain. In a harsh primitive world, the instinct for pleasure enabled us to persevere. As the brain developed new and more complex layers, humans acquired the capacity to think, speak, and scientists speculate, to experience happiness.

A specific area in our post "caveman" brain known as the left pre-frontal cortex—located just above the left eye—appears to be one of the brain's H-spot, the locus of "happiness."[6]

Where our culture locates the source of happiness is another matter. Too often, TV, film and glossy magazines present happiness as leading the "Lifestyles of the Rich and Famous." Of course, one only need watch an episode of the "Real Housewives" to witness that purchasing a sports car, designer gown or mansion does not guarantee happiness!

So why do so many of us seek pleasure over happiness? It's what our society tells us to do. Just turn on the TV, go online, or drive down your street. We are bombarded with commercials, billboards and movies that reinforce the falsehood that money and materialism will make us happy.

Consumer culture and conspicuous consumption may boost the economy, but it doesn't boost our happiness. As I noted earlier: "No external conditions are required for your happiness. Happiness is who you truly are."

A helpful way to distinguish pleasure from happiness is to think of money versus abundance. We tend to view money in the same way we regard pleasure. We continually seek more of it. Just as relentless pleasure seeking can prevent us from experiencing authentic happiness, an insatiable desire for money

pleasure = specific

prevents us from experiencing authentic abundance. That's a topic for an entirely separate book!

Happiness can certainly be influenced by external situations and circumstances in our life: a beautiful home, a good education or a loving family, but genuine happiness can flourish within us independently of any of these. Pleasure, on the other hand, is entirely dependent on a specific experience, at a specific time and specific place.

There are many people who are content going through life pursuing pleasure. Trust me, I used to be that person.

There is nothing wrong with enjoying pleasure. It is wired into our biology. The problem happens when seeking pleasure becomes a way of life. Too often our search for pleasure is a form of escapism, a coping mechanism or addiction that eventually sabotages our happiness.

Pleasure can often mask itself as happiness. But pull off that mask and pleasure can look a lot like depression. I find that a common theme among many of my private clients is the constant seeking of pleasure as a strategy to avoid dealing with other issues. Have you noticed how many people—whether in your own life or on Reality TV—self-medicate their sadness with pleasure?

Can eating an entire bag of chocolate cookies really bring you deep happiness when you're feeling sad? Can a relationship only based on sexual pleasure foster long-term happiness? Can waiting in line all night to purchase a newer and slightly more sophisticated version of your phone, truly make you a happier person?

While, again, there is nothing wrong with cookies, sex or technology, if you desire an authentic, fulfilling and joyful life, it's time for a new strategy.

First we must unravel what motivates our choices? The solution can be surprisingly simple. The key is to ask oneself: "Is the choice I'm making satisfying a short-term desire or fostering my long-term happiness?"

I'm the first to admit that choosing a life of happiness over pleasure isn't easy. We often don't go with the choice that we intuitively know is good for us. Often this is because the right choice isn't always the easiest choice.

When you make conscious choices aligned with your inner "happiness compass," the path that was once obscure becomes clearer. What I find fascinating is that even small choices help us to retrain and restructure the brain. Each time you choose an apple instead of a Hershey's bar if you wish to lose weight or resist the purchase of yet another pair of designer shoes if you already have a closet of them, you're creating new brain pathways.

The more you exercise your will on a regular basis when choosing happiness over pleasure, the easier it will be when you are faced with more challenging choices such as whether to leave a relationship or break out on a new career path.

Why? Because, you've already created the neural pathways in your brain to make it happen! How do athletes prepare for a marathon or a big sporting event? Regular and consistent practice! We train our brain in the exact same way.

I've seen this work over and over again not only for myself but for my corporate clients and students. The reason this works is because of what scientists refer to as neuroplasticity. Each time we make the choice to pursue authentic happiness over short-term pleasure it becomes less of a struggle, in fact, eventually such behavior becomes effortless and automatic.

Choosing a life exclusively focused on self-gratification may be the easier and simpler path, but the road that leads to happiness is far richer. Trust me, I've taken both. I know.

Happiness is not about giving up the path of pleasure. It's the conscious choice of moving from a life enslaved to pleasure to a life of fulfillment and purpose.

There's a fork in the road in front of you. You get to decide which path to take.

↓ grateful for things right now.

↓ gratitude social benefit

↓ 1 thing you're grateful for.

Secret 3 | If You Want To Get Happy, Practice Gratitude!

In order for you to continue receiving abundance in the future, you have to express gratitude for the abundance manifesting in the present. –Dr. Jay Kumar

What's one thing you're grateful for that happened to you today?

Among all the emotions humans are capable of expressing, brain scans show us that gratitude appears to be the one that most easily and instantly makes us feel happy!

This astonishing discovery appears to be related to the vast network in the brain known as *mirror neurons*. Among all the major breakthroughs to have come out from neuroscience in the past decade, in my opinion, the discovery of mirror neurons tops the chart!

Do you ever wonder why it is that when you see others laughing and smiling, you feel the urge to smile or laugh? Or when you watch a spider crawl up someone's arm, you get the same creepy feeling as if it were happening to you? That's because of the brain's mirror neurons

Even though you're only seeing the action, the same neurons in your brain fire as if you were having the experience yourself. A healthy and normal brain mirrors the activity of what it sees in the world.

Mirror neurons induce the human quality of empathy. When we see someone fall, our first reaction is to go and check if the person is okay. It's a built-in response in the human brain to feel another person's joy, sadness, exuberance

mirror neurons :)

or grief. The brain is constantly mirroring whatever actions it observes.

Mirror neurons are the reason human beings have the capacity to experience compassion or express love. Scientists speculate that our ancestors would never have survived in the harsh brutal world had it not been for the development of mirror neurons. Prior to the development of language, the human brain had to recognize and interpret meaning to non-verbal cues—the difference between a smile and a snarl—to gauge the mood and feelings of others.

If the human brain weren't wired to express empathy, scientists suggest our species might not have acquired the ability for cooperation, sharing, nurturing and bonding, the prerequisites for civilization.

Contrary to what we might see or read in the media, the human brain is wired for empathy, compassion, love and gratitude. The key to humanity's survival may well reside in our mirror neurons. Where would we be if people didn't come together in times of hunger, disaster or strife?

Mirror neurons are the reason we cry when we watch a sad film, rejoice when we hear uplifting news, wince when we witness someone in pain, or chuckle when we watch puppies play. Mirror neurons allow us to feel what it is like to walk in someone else's shoes.

Interestingly, not everyone's mirror neurons are equally developed. While not conclusive, some recent studies propose that Asperger's syndrome and autism may be linked to mirror neuron dysfunction.[7]

Science shows that it isn't just humans who have mirror neurons. Current research suggests that only five known species on the planet possess a developed mirror neuron system—all higher primates, such as apes and chimps, elephants, dolphins and dogs. And people!

Why are mirror neurons so important? Expressing gratitude helps us build our "empathy muscles."

Here are a few more reasons why gratitude promotes health and happiness:

1. A 2003 study at the University of Miami had college students keep a daily journal of things for which they felt grateful.[8] The other test group was assigned to keep a journal of what annoyed them. Those who kept gratitude journals were found to have an overall improvement in enthusiasm, determination and energy compared to those in the test group. Even doing this exercise once a week, rather than daily, brought similar benefits.

2. The same University of Miami researchers revealed two more amazing discoveries. People who wrote in their gratitude journals experienced positive changes in behavior such as an increased desire to exercise. What really impressed the researchers is that practicing gratitude appeared to promote overall health and reduce the feeling of physical pain!

3. Feeling sad and can't sleep? Practice more gratitude. A 2012 study at the University of Hong Kong examined the sleep patterns of people suffering from depression.[9] The results were startling. The group that practiced gratitude exercises benefitted not only from greater sleep, but also less frequent episodes of depression.

4. A 2009 study by the National Institutes of Health placed participants in fMRI machines to measure blood flow in the brain.[10] The volunteers were told to engender feelings of gratitude. Those participants who felt the emotion of gratitude experienced more activity in the brain's hypothalamus than those in the test group who did not. An active hypothalamus is helpful since it regulates sleep, digestion, and metabolism and can help to mitigate stress.

Gratitude has a powerful social benefit. It helps us to feel more connected to others. Just saying the simple words "Thank you" can lift us out of our own individual concerns and serve to remind us of the joy and happiness that others bring to in our life. Expressing gratitude not only benefits the recipient of our appreciation, but oneself.

Try it out for yourself. Say "Thank you" to *five* different people every day for *five* consecutive days. Embody a genuine feeling of gratitude as you do so, perhaps even offering a smile to that person. After the fifth day notice how you feel. Chances are, you'll experience a remarkable boost of inner happiness.

Again, this isn't magic, its real science. So, how exactly does gratitude make us happy?

When we express gratitude, it's as if the brain immediately stepped on the "emotional brakes" and suddenly, the emotions of sadness, self-pity or stress that were driving us, are slowed.

From the perspective of neuroscience, another part of the brain that fires when we express thanks is the left pre-frontal cortex, a region just above our left eye that brain scans correlate with feelings of contentment, meaning and self-worth.

In the "Happiness" course I co-teach every year, we have students perform a variety of "gratitude-building" exercises throughout the semester. Here are two simple and easy-to-use gratitude tools that you can incorporate into your daily regimen.

1. Bring to mind *five* people—alive or deceased—whom you are genuinely grateful for in your life. They don't have to be the same five people every day you do this. They don't even have to be people. You can think of a pet, the one you have now or the one you loved as a child. The important thing is that you do this exercise the first thing when you wake up! Envision each person in your mind for about 10-15 seconds, and send either a verbal or silent affirmation expressing why that person—or dog or cat—mattered to you. The other important thing is to not only engage your thoughts, but the *feeling* of gratitude. You'll be surprised by how much this morning exercise will brighten your day.

2. Another effective and simple tool is to create a short list of *five* memories when you felt genuine happiness. Your list might include the day you married, the birth of a child, the day you graduated college, or appreciation for your health or prosperity. Print out several copies of this list and place them by your bed, at your office, on your bathroom mirror or take a snapshot of it so you can view the list on your smartphone. Each time you look at the list, repeat out loud to yourself *one* different item on the list that evokes a feeling of gratitude. Again, don't just state the item, feel it!

I've been regularly doing these exercises myself for the past two years, and what a difference they've made in my life. My students and clients report back to me in amazement at how something so fundamental and easy as expressing gratitude has deepened their ability to feel happy. It affirms the innate power we each have to feel joy.

Just as we lift weights to build muscle, neuroscience affirms that our brain is a muscle that can be trained and developed. As we cultivate gratitude we automatically experience greater enthusiasm and contentment.

As the Sufi poet Rumi put it: "Gratitude is the wine for the soul. Go on. Get drunk."

Brain fatigue

Secret 4 | The Great Outdoors: Nature's Natural Spa

Nature doesn't come with a built-in Wi-Fi signal, but you're guaranteed to have a strong connection! –Dr. Jay Kumar

Do you chronically feel stressed, depressed, or lethargic? If so, it might be the result of a condition informally termed, brain fatigue.

Do any of the following situations sound familiar? The alarm jolts you out of sleep at 6 a.m. You wake up feeling exhausted but counter it with a jolt of caffeine. You quickly shower, dress, scarf down breakfast, and rush to school or work only to stew in traffic.

You already feel pressure and you haven't even arrived at the office yet. Work deadlines make it a burger or taco with a soft drink at your desk. By late afternoon, you're slamming more coffee or biting into something sweet just to get through the day. If you do make it to the gym, it's lifting weights or running on the treadmill to a loud playlist. Finally home, you feel spent and try to unwind with some TV or checking Facebook. Though exhausted, you turn in but can't seem to fall asleep. Your brain is still racing from the chaos and tumult of your day.

If much of this resembles your life, you're not alone.

Here's a startling fact. In our modern, 24/7 high-tech world, the average person's brain is bombarded with the equivalent of 174 newspapers of data every day![11] That's some five times the amount of sensory information a person received just 30 years ago. No wonder many of us experience the harmful impact of brain-fatigue. As individuals and a society we feel exhausted, overwhelmed and stressed on a daily basis.

Even when we seek to "unwind" we end up feeling more tightly wound. As individuals and as a culture we take pride and boast of our "busy lives." Once home, we can't quit our e-habit. Even in our bedrooms, living rooms, even bathrooms, we peruse our screens, feeling the need to check email, Facebook, Twitter or Instagram.

Perhaps on the weekend you head out with buddies to "relax" over a few drinks. But nowadays sports bars too have a half dozen or more big screen TVs, each broadcasting the current big game. Outings with friends soon devolve into sensory overload. You visit the mall and are hit with perfumes, busy food courts, and tens of thousands of outfits, purses, toys and shoes.

We even cram our vacations with activity. Small wonder we feel depleted once we return home. Soon, we find ourselves requiring a holiday to recover from our holidays.

Is it any wonder so many of us struggle to fall asleep? Insomnia is on the rise, so too numerous varieties of anxiety and mood disorders. Studies show the toll is highest among those of us who live in cities. A McGill University study shows that people who live in major urban centers have a 20% greater risk of anxiety and nearly a 40% risk of mood-disorders.[12]

When study participants were put into fMRI machines and shown images of hectic urban life, the area of the brain, known as the *amygdala*, showed greater activity. This is the area of the brain that governs the "fight-or-flight response." When this mechanism runs rampant, we experience heightened levels of stress and anxiety.

But let me offer this bit of good news! A powerful and natural antidote to stress may be just outside your window—it's called Mother Nature!

Some researchers suggest the reason that stress has become the malady of modern life and that we suffer from brain-fatigue is the result of "Nature-Deficit Disorder."[13] Never heard of it? A growing body of research proposes that we as a society are becoming more and more disconnected from the healing power of nature.

Why do you think spas play soundtracks of chirping birds, babbling brooks and breaking waves? The brain immediately feels soothed and lulled into harmony by such natural sounds.

It's not only nature's chirps and rustlings that soothe our stress. Simply spending time in nature soothes our soul. A short walk in the woods; watching a sunset; stopping to take in a hummingbird as it darts between flowers, each of these experiences in nature quiet the brain.

Consider the outdoors as your free spa. A few minutes of stillness can place your brain into an alpha-wave state, as if you'd just come home from a weekend at a five-star health resort.

Nature, it turns out, is your brain's best friend!

While religion and spirituality have always extolled the glory and healing potential of nature, science—specifically from the field of neuroscience—is preaching the same message.

In the same experiment outlined above, when participants were shown images of the outdoors, activity in the anterior cingulate, the area of the brain that governs altruism, contentment and an overall sense of peace, flashed with activity.

So how exactly does nature heal? The answer resides in our brains and relates again to the concept known as the *relaxation response*, a mechanism wired into our biology to cope with stress.

Another emerging field, known as eco-psychology, advocates that though the human brain may be adapting to our fast-paced world, its original function was to respond to the natural world in which we dwelled and evolved over millennia.

According to this area of study, human beings have an instinctual need to connect with nature, something known as *nature connectedness*, a concept originally developed in the last century by the biologist Edward O. Wilson.

This evolutionary connection to nature activates the part of the brain known as the *insula*, the area that governs our internal feelings and sensations. The insula gauges how we feel and what we experience. It also helps us to enter the present moment.

Science shows that nature is sometimes the best medicine. Dr. Ulrich at the Center for Health Research and Design published one of the earliest studies in 1984 in the journal *Science*. He observed that patients recovering from surgery healed more quickly and required less pain medication when placed in hospital rooms with views of nature, versus those in rooms facing buildings.

Ulrich concluded that when people are immersed in nature, the brain automatically eases into the passive attention-mode that is connected with the healing alpha wave brain state.

This doesn't require ditching Los Angeles or London for Maui. Research suggests that even a short 10-15 minute walk in the park during one's lunch break, touching—hugging is even better—a tree on your walk to the office, or "stopping to smell the roses" are all beneficial.

These benefits accrue to adults as well as children. Indeed, it's not just adults who feel stressed. In my years of teaching at university, I sadly see far too many of my students feeling overwhelmed by stress, anxiety and agitation. In a study of children diagnosed with ADHD at the University of Illinois, children with ADHD were divided into three randomized groups. One group was led on a 20-minute walk in a park, another in a residential neighborhood and the third group down a busy urban street. After each walk, the children were given the same cognitive test to measure memory, focus and concentration.

You can probably guess which group performed best on the test? That's right, the children who had walked in the park. Even more intriguing is that the children were told not to take any prescription medication for their ADHD on the day of the experiment. The study showed that a "dose of nature" worked just as well, if not better, than a dose of medication.

The findings, later presented in a 2004 article of the *American Journal of Public Health*, suggest that our environment—for better or worse—affects our health and happiness.[14]

But can a short walk in the park truly provide scientifically measurable benefits to a healthy adult? According to a fascinating 2013 study from researchers at University of Edinburgh, published in the *British Journal of Sports Medicine*[15], the answer is yes! Just as in the study with children with ADHD, adults were sent on a 30-minute walk in three distinct Edinburgh neighborhoods. Each participant strolled through the historic town center, then through a large park and lastly along a busy downtown thoroughfare.

On their walk, each participant wore a portable wireless neural-imaging headset that mapped his or her brain waves in real-time.

The results were clear. The brief walk in the park induced a calming alpha state in the brain waves of participants. The next time you feel fatigue or stress, one quick—and free—solution is to spend time in nature. Hey, Henry David Thoreau knew what he was talking about.

The benefits of this type of self-healing apply across the board. Nature has the power to bestow calm, clarity and contentment and can boost our immune system.

As the renowned writer Jane Austen put it: "To sit in the shade on a fine day and look upon verdure is the most perfect refreshment."

If you've been putting off relaxing because you think it requires the expense of a massage or visit to a spa, think again. You may find the same benefits from a short walk along a lake, a tree-lined street or during a romp in the park with your pooch.

Secret 5 | An LSD Trip for the Soul: Laughing, Singing & Dancing

My one sure trick to get happy, a healthy dose of LSD: Laughing, Singing and Dancing! —Dr. Jay Kumar

Health Is A Laughing Matter

We've all heard the expression, "Laughter is the best medicine." Well, it's official! Studies affirm that this is absolutely true. Whether your laughter comes from watching Homer Simpson, Jon Stewart or Tina Fey, no matter—it's all good for your health.

Numerous studies affirm that laughter boosts the immune system, helps to alleviate pain and strengthens the heart. Such benefits are amplified when laughter is shared.

Here are five reasons why it's good to laugh.

1. Laughter decreases stress by producing more of your body's "natural killer" cells. These cells are a type of white blood cell, shown to assist in the prevention of cancer, HIV and other threats to our immune system.

2. A 2005 University of Maryland study showed that a good dose of mirth helps to regulate blood pressure and enhances cardiovascular health.[16] Laughter also appears to expand the linings in our blood vessels, improving blood flow and oxygenation in the circulatory system.

3. How about going on a laughter diet? Laughing a 100 times is the equivalent of 10 to 15 minutes of aerobic exercise. So the next time you can't make it to the gym, catch an episode of your favorite sitcom and enjoy a laugh workout instead.

4. Next time you're in pain, your best prescription may be a punch line. In his autobiography "Anatomy of an Illness," Norman Cousins wrote about his experience of using laughter as an effective way to alleviate the physical pain of a crippling and debilitating illness. Medical studies show that laughter releases endorphins, our body's natural morphine, briefly increasing our body's tolerance for pain.

5. Move over, multivitamins and green tea! Laughter is shown to have a powerful benefit to our overall immune system. Studies indicate that laughing increases levels of immunoglobulin A, an important antibody in human saliva that fights infection, and also produces interferon, proteins in the body that combat harmful pathogens in our immune system.[17]

Mark Twain summed it up perfectly: *"Against the assault of laughter nothing can stand."*

So if a joke you tell falls flat, tell the listener to thank you anyway, because you just boosted her health. Speaking of friends, thank you to my friend and radio host Doug Stephan for turning me on to the idea that LSD is the perfect acronym for what all of us need more of in our lives: Laughing, Singing and Dancing!

The Brain Is Alive with the Sound of Music

Archeology tells us that music has been around for millennia. It's only in the past decade, however, that neuroscience has explored how music enhances our health and happiness.[18]

One reason so many of us love live concerts or listening to a favorite vocalist, band or orchestra is because music affects the reward and pleasure centers in the brain by releasing dopamine, the chemical that governs our emotional wants and desires.

While listening to music is helpful, singing is even better. Researchers at Harvard Medical School reason that it rewires damaged areas of the brain, a breakthrough they uncovered while helping stroke victims regain the ability to speak.

Speaking and singing are human activities that occur in two different areas of the brain. By putting their words to song, stroke patients with speech impairments were able to use the "singing centers" of the brain to retrain the damaged "speech centers."

The same principle appears to work in the brains of people who stutter. It's why in the film, "The King's Speech," we see King George VI, told by his speech therapist, to sing the words of his addresses to the British people, before delivering them.

Even if you don't stutter or suffer from a stroke, singing has a number of positive benefits. For starters, singing improves memory. Did you ever wonder why it's easier to recall the lyrics to a favorite song than a random 10-digit phone number?

There appears to be an intimate connection in the brain between singing and memory. A structure deep in the brain, known as the hippocampus, is where new memories are stored. Activities such as singing and playing a musical instrument

Boost memory

promote healthy functioning of this area of the brain. This is also good news for people suffering from dementia or Alzheimer's. More hospitals and nursing homes are using the power of song to help in the treatment of these illnesses.

But you don't have to be a researcher at Harvard to know that singing new information helps us retain it. Singing is how most of us learned to memorize the alphabet. The next time you need to remember the name of a new client, try singing her name a few times in your head and see if that helps.

Not only does singing boost memory and prevent the risk of Alzheimer's disease, it is also a surefire way to lift our spirits and ward off depression. It also can help reduce stress. The limbic system—emotional region of the brain—is positively affected by singing.

Just as with laughter, singing with others boosts its effectiveness. No doubt this is why when we sing with others whether in a chorus, at a rock concert or at synagogue or church, we feel joyous and alive. So even if you're like me and can't carry a tune if your life depended on it, go ahead and sing. It's good for you.

I have to agree with Ella Fitzgerald, who voiced it best: "The only thing better than singing is more singing."

The Groove Is In the Brain

Whether it's salsa, swing, tap or tango, dancing is the key to a long and healthy life.

That's precisely the finding of a 20-year study published in the *New England Journal of Medicine*.[19] The long-term study of senior citizens set out to ascertain if physical activities and cognitive activities, such as reading, doing crossword puzzles, writing or playing a musical instrument diminished the risk of Alzheimer's disease. What they found was stunning.

Of all the activities, both cognitive and physical, dancing had the highest ability to reduce the risk of dementia and Alzheimer's disease. How much so? People who reported to dance regularly had a 76% reduced chance of cognitive impairment! Here's why.

Scientists believe that dancing had one thing that differentiated it from other activities in the study. Dancing uses more areas of our brain's memory and learning centers than other activities. When we dance, we simultaneously integrate several brain functions: movement, emotion, music, thinking, sight, touch and hearing.

In essence, people who dance are building a bigger "cognitive reserve" in their brains than those who don't. The more cognitive capital we accumulate, the more our brains remain healthy and strong.

Like with laughter and singing, dance is an effective antidote to stress and depression. Dancing regulates our mood by stimulating the hippocampus, and releases endorphins to boost our spirits. Dancing also doubles the brain's blood and oxygen levels, all of which are great for achieving health and happiness.

While dancing has benefits in the short-term for regulating our mood and emotions, it's the long-term impact of dance on memory and brain health that are garnering attention.

Now you possess several steps toward health and happiness worth taking! So whatever form of LSD you choose—laughing, singing or dancing—you really can't go wrong.

In the "moving" words of the famous choreographer Martha Graham: "Dance is the hidden language of the soul of the body."

Do you know what I really love about laughter, song, and dance? These are pursuits shared by every person on the planet, regardless of religion, politics, class or culture. I love travel and no matter how remote the country or foreign the culture, I've always found people enjoying each of these pursuits. If there's a universal language, it must be laughter, song and dance.

Works Cited

1   "Think Twice: How the Gut's 'Second Brain' Influences Mood and Well-Being" *Scientific American* February 12, 2010. http://www.scientificamerican.com/article.cfm?id=gut-second-brain

2   "Stress the Killer Disease" *Psychology Today* Nov. 2012. http://www.psychologytoday.com/blog/evolutionary-psychiatry/201211/stress-the-killer-disease

3   "Accelerated telomere shortening in response to life stress" Proceedings of the National Academy of Sciences Dec. 2004. http://www.ncbi.nlm.nih.gov/pubmed/15574496

4   "Yoga for Anxiety & Depression" *Harvard Health Publications* April 2009. http://www.health.harvard.edu/newsletters/Harvard_Mental_Health_Letter/2009/April/Yoga-for-anxiety-and-depression

5   http://www.semel.ucla.edu/cousins/research/mind-body-interactions

6   "The Role of the Brain in Happiness" *Psychology Today* Feb. 2013. http://www.psychologytoday.com/blog/in-the-face-adversity/201302/the-role-the-brain-in-happiness

7   "Mirror Neurons and Autism" http://www.autism-help.org/points-mirror-neurons.htm

8   "Counting Blessings Versus Burdens: An Experimental Investigation of Gratitude and Subjective Well-Being in Daily Life" *Journal of Personality and Social Psychology*, 2003, Vol. 84, No. 2, 377–389. http://www.stybelpeabody.com/newsite/pdf/gratitude.pdf

9   "The Differential Effects of Gratitude and Sleep on Psychological Distress in Patients with Chronic Pain" *Journal of Health Psychology* March 2012. http://hpq.sagepub.com/content/early/2012/03/12/1359105312439733.abstract

10   "The Grateful Brain" *Psychology Today* Nov. 2012. http://www.psychologytoday.com/blog/prefrontal-nudity/201211/the-grateful-brain

11   "Hit the Reset Button in Your Brain" *New York Times* Aug. 2014. http://www.nytimes.com/2014/08/10/opinion/sunday/hit-the-reset-button-in-your-brain.html

12   "Researchers Find Higher Mental Illness Among City Dwellers" *Voice of America*. http://www.voanews.com/content/researchers-find-higher-mental-illness-among-city-dwellers-124386509/171515.html

13   "Connecting With Nature Boosts Creativity and Health" *National Geographic* June 2013. http://news.nationalgeographic.com/news/2013/06/130628-richard-louv-nature-deficit-disorder-health-environment/

14   "A Potential Natural Treatment for Attention-Deficit/Hyperactivity Disorder: Evidence From a National Study" *Am J Public Health*. 2004 September; 94(9): 1580–1586. http://www.ncbi.nlm.nih.gov/pmc/articles/PMC1448497/

15   "The urban brain: analysing outdoor physical activity with mobile EEG" *Br J Sports Med* doi:10.1136/

bjsports-2012-091877. http://bjsm.bmj.com/content/
early/2013/03/05/bjsports-2012-091877.abstract

16   "University Of Maryland School Of Medicine
Study Shows Laughter Helps Blood Vessels Function Better" *Science Daily* March 2005. http://www.sciencedaily.com/
releases/2005/03/050309111444.htm

17   "Humor and Laughter May Influence Health IV.
Humor and Immune Function" *Evidence Based Complementary
Alternative Medicine* June 2009; 6(2): 159–164. http://www.
ncbi.nlm.nih.gov/pmc/articles/PMC2686627/

18   "Why Music Makes Our Brain Sing" *The New York
Times* March 2013. http://www.nytimes.com/2013/06/09/
opinion/sunday/why-music-makes-our-brain-sing.
html?_r=2&

19   "Dancing Your Way to Better Health" *WebMD*
http://www.webmd.com/fitness-exercise/features/
dancing-your-way-to-better-health

Acknowledgments

The *Brain, Body & Being*™ book would not be possible without the tremendous encouragement and faith from my dearest friends, family and colleagues.

Gali Kronenberg's meticulous eye, insightful comments and talent for translating my ideas into succinct, clear prose, immeasurably enriched my book. I especially wish to thank the invaluable efforts by Lori Brown, Greg French, Michael Gardiner and Don Zyck for their guidance and unwavering support in this project.

I also appreciate the illuminating insights of my academic colleagues Dr. Gail Stearns, Dr. Menas Kafatos and Dr. Michael Irwin.

Big Shout Out to my amazing "online family" at Live Happy LLC for helping spread the global happiness movement.

Lastly, many thanks to all my students at Loyola Marymount University and Chapman University who continue to teach and inspire me to manifest my full potential both in and out of the classroom.

About Dr. Jay Kumar

As a renowned thought leader and public speaker, Dr. Jay Kumar expertly counsels organizations and businesses on harnessing the art and science of happiness for both short- and long-term success.

Clients across the globe—from lean start-ups to large corporations—have benefited from his highly effective, easy-to-learn and scientifically proven insights and techniques. In addition to consulting businesses and individuals, Dr. Jay stays at the forefront of brain research as a respected university professor.

He holds a Ph.D. in cognitive science and religious studies from the California Institute of Integral Studies and an M.A. in international political economy and a concentration in international business from Columbia University. He has also pursued advanced graduate studies at Georgetown University and UCLA.

Stay Connected, Share the Health & Happiness

If you enjoyed and benefitted from the wealth of helpful tools presented here, stay engaged with the *Brain, Body & Being*™ community and learn more about Dr. Jay Kumar by visiting www.DrJayKumar.com or by connecting on Facebook & Twitter -@docjaykumar.